D0055858

This Music Guidebook is part of a diverse collection of
music and knowledge available at Blue Marble Music

deep sleep 101

MUSIC AND GUIDEBOOK

FOR A GOOD NIGHT'S SLEEP

Blue Marble, Inc. 205 Brazos Street Austin, TX 78701

www.bluemarblemusic.com email: info@bluemarblemusic.com

deep sleep 101

MUSIC AND GUIDEBOOK

FOR A GOOD NIGHT'S SLEEP

BY GREGG D. JACOBS, PH.D.

www.bluemarblemusic.com 1/800-860-9442

A WORD FROM OUR
FOUNDER

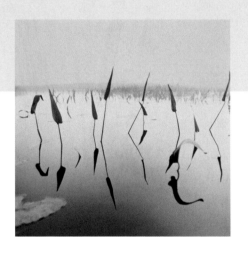

Every once in awhile things come together, flowing naturally from casual coincidence. Such is the case with this book.

As we began designing Blue Marble's Music Guidebook Collection, we discussed many ideas with customers all around the world. Everywhere we turned, busy adults were complaining about "poor sleep". We thought music might help, so we started working on a relaxing music CD and a quick reference guide to improving sleep.

We wanted the very best sleep advice for this project, so we contacted Dr. Gregg Jacobs at Harvard Medical School. Coincidentally, Dr. Jacobs, author of *Say Good Night to Insomnia*, was just finishing up a study of music's effect on brainwaves, relaxation and sleep. The preliminary results from his study confirmed our instincts – music *can* enhance relaxation and sleep.

With guidance from Dr. Jacobs, our music experts put together a music collection that will help quiet your mind, relax your body and prepare you for sleep. (By the way, our baby twins at home have yet to stay awake through the second song!)

Deep Sleep 101 is part of a Collection of Music Guidebooks that brings our customers a broad, diverse collection of music and knowledge. May the knowledge you discover and the music you hear enrich your life. That is our goal at Blue Marble.

Steve Stone, Founder
Blue Marble, L.L.C.

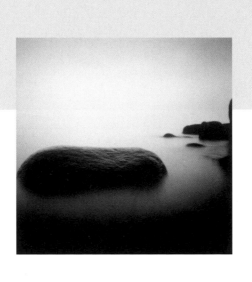

GUIDEBOOK
OUTLINE

MUSIC AND THE
BRAIN

section 1

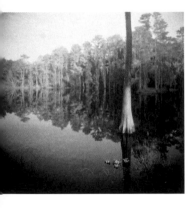

MUSIC, THE BRAIN AND SLEEP

As humans evolved over millions of years, music was tightly woven into the lives of virtually every culture around the globe. Recent scientific research is beginning to show that music is part of our biological makeup, encoded in our genes as part of what makes us human.

We recently completed a study at Harvard Medical School that tested music's effect on the brain. We also compared the effectiveness of listening to music against the effectiveness of meditation for relaxing the brain and the body.

The results show that listening to relaxing music can produce theta brainwaves that are similar to those in deep relaxation and stage 1 sleep. In fact, data from the study suggests that, for half of the people studied, music was as effective as meditation in producing these relaxation brainwaves.

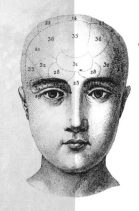

Listening to ●
certain types
of relaxing
music
increases
slow theta
brainwaves
that are
similar to
those
involved in
deep relax-
ation and
Stage 1
sleep.

HOW MUSIC WORKS

Music exerts its therapeutic, relaxing effects in several ways:

z *Music absorbs our attention and distracts our thoughts away from worries and concerns.*

z *Music acts as a repetitive mental stimulus that provides constant input into the sensory receptors and brain, which lowers arousal and induces relaxation.*

z *Music can evoke recent personal memories of pleasure and may even evoke ancient memories within your DNA of pleasure experienced by your ancestors.*

THE BIG

PICTURE

section 2

THE SILENT EPIDEMIC

Sleep is a highly complex restoration process for the mind and the body. The average person today spends roughly 23 years of a 75-year lifespan asleep. Despite these facts, extensive study of sleep is really just getting underway.

When a person experiences chronic poor sleep, health and well-being can suffer significantly. With surveys now showing that half of the adult U.S. population experiences sleep difficulties, it is clear that sleep disorders have reached epidemic status.

LIFESTYLE DE-EVOLUTION

The reason underlying such a widespread problem with sleep is simple. We have evolved into lifestyles that create an imbalanced system in our minds and bodies.

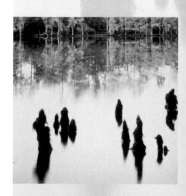

A NEW APPROACH

Fifteen years of research on relaxation and sleep at Harvard Medical School has given me pretty clear insight into the core issues involved in sleep and a keen understanding of what works in treating sleep difficulties. Research suggests that the only effective way to cure insomnia is by re-training the mind and the body to produce the physiological changes that enhance sleep.

These changes cannot be made with sleeping pills, quick-fix gimmicks or herbal remedies. It usually takes a change in lifestyle or specific behaviors to effectively change sleep patterns.

To test this approach, we created a drug-free insomnia program at Harvard Medical School. Of the patients treated with this program, 100 percent reported improved sleep.

The success of the drug-free program stems from its focus on the mind/body causes of poor sleep, rather than treating surface-level symptoms with drugs and chemicals.

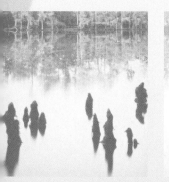

OUR GENETIC HERITAGE

Our human evolution over millions of years required a variety of daily behaviors essential to good sleep. These behaviors included:

z *Regular physical activity for hunting, gathering food, planting and harvesting*

z *Exposure to physical stressors (such as predators) that involved fighting or fleeing*

z *Eating all-natural foods that contained no synthetic chemicals*

z *Regular exposure to daily and seasonal cycles of light, darkness, quiet, solitude and nature*

Because these behaviors were part of our evolution over millions of years, they became part of our genetic make-up and deep, ancestral memories in the brain.

OUR NEW SOW LIFESTYLE

In a remarkably short period of time, we have dramatically altered our lifestyle. We have become sedentary office workers (SOWs) with 'evolved' lifestyles that do not provide us the basic stimuli that our minds and bodies need to be healthy. For example:

z *Instead of regular physical activity, we sit for hours at a time at the office and at home*

z *Our minds experience an overload of chronic psychological stressors as we negotiate complex social, family and work structures*

z *We have very little exposure to sunlight*

z *Rather than experiencing silence, we constantly listen to radio, television and telephones*

z *We tend to eat processed foods that contain high doses of non-natural chemicals*

To sleep effectively, we must reestablish a few of the behaviors from our evolutionary heritage.

BASICS OF
SLEEP

music has charms

This guidebook for improving sleep culminates with a list of techniques that will likely cause significant improvements in your sleep. To understand why focus is placed on these specific techniques, it is helpful to first understand a few basics about sleep.

to soothe a savage

breast, to soften

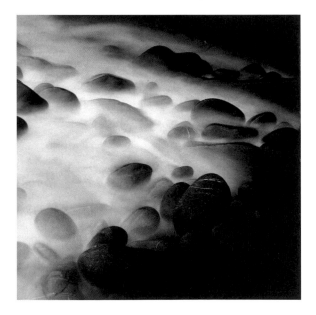

rocks, or bend

a knotted oak.

- william congreve

THE CYCLICAL PATTERN OF SLEEP

During a night's sleep, we move from Stage 1 to Stage 4 and then to Rapid Eye Movement (REM) sleep in about 90 minutes. We move through four to six of these 90-minute sleep cycles during the night, spending about 5 percent of the night in Stage 1, 50 percent in Stage 2, 20 percent in deep sleep and 25 percent in REM sleep. Sleep consistently follows this cyclical pattern.

Early in the night, deep-sleep periods are lengthier and can sometimes last up to one hour, whereas REM periods last only a few minutes. Later in the night, however, deep-sleep periods grow shorter and the duration of REM periods increase to as much as one hour by the final sleep cycle. Consequently, we obtain most of our deep sleep during the first half of the night, and the majority of our dream sleep in the second half.

● **Dream** on.

Most common **dream** theme - falling.

Most common nightmare theme - being chased.

A thunderstorm stimulates **dream**ing.

Almost everyone **dream**s in color.

Babies **dream** in utero.

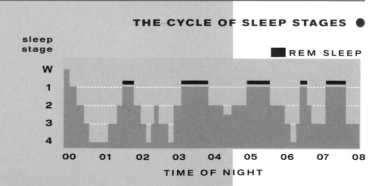

THE CYCLE OF SLEEP STAGES ●

sleep stage

■ REM SLEEP

W
1
2
3
4

00   01   02   03   04   05   06   07   08

TIME OF NIGHT

BODY-TEMPERATURE RHYTHMS

Although you may believe that your body temperature remains constant at about 98.6° F, it actually follows a circadian ("about a day") rhythm that varies throughout the day.

Body temperature is lowest in the early morning hours and then begins to rise. It continues to increase until attaining its daily peak around 6:00 p.m. A few hours later, body temperature drops until we fall asleep, then declines more rapidly until it reaches its daily low again at about 4:00 a.m. In a healthy young adult, the variation between the daily minimum and maximum body temperature is about 1.5 degrees.

● BODY TEMPERATURE AND THE SLEEP/WAKE CYCLE

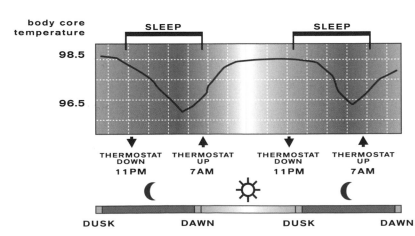

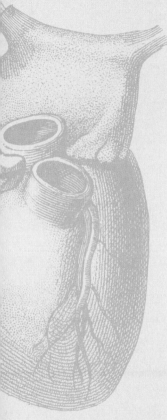

STAGES OF SLEEP

Stage 1 During a typical night's sleep, we close our eyes and first spend a few minutes in a state of relaxed wakefulness that is characterized by a brainwave pattern named alpha. In this state our thoughts gradually wander and our bodies begin to relax. Next, we drift into Stage 1 sleep, which is a drowsy, transitional state between waking and sleeping where your: muscles relax; respiration and heart rate slows; and a slower brainwave pattern called "theta" is generated. Stage 1 sleep is often described as "dreamy", "floating", "wondering" and "losing a direct train of thought".

Stage 2 Following a few minutes in Stage 1, we enter into Stage 2. This is deeper than Stage 1, since we are more detached from the outside world. Stage 2 sleep is characterized by brainwave patterns called sleep spindles and K-complexes and is regarded as a light stage of sleep, for we are awakened easily from it.

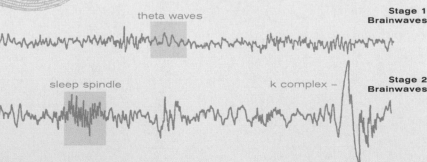

theta waves

Stage 1 Brainwaves

sleep spindle

k complex –

Stage 2 Brainwaves

Stages 3 and 4 (Deep Sleep)

After about 45 minutes in Stage 2, we enter deep sleep, called Stages 3 and 4, which is distinguished by very slow brainwave patterns named "delta". During deep sleep, our physiological activity – including respiration, oxygen consumption, heart rate, and blood pressure – realizes its lowest level of the day. It is very difficult to awaken from deep sleep.

The Purpose of Deep Sleep – Physical Regeneration

Deep sleep seems to serve a major biological restorative function by shutting down the brain and the body and renewing our physical energy. During deep sleep, our immune system turns on to combat illnesses, which may explain why we seem to sleep more when we are ill.

Research suggests that deep sleep is essential and represents the most important stage for the restoration of our physical bodies.

Stage 3 & 4 (Deep Sleep) Brainwaves

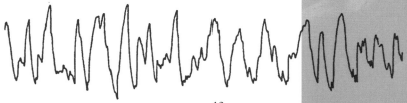

REM SLEEP

After about 45 minutes in deep sleep, we return to Stage 2 for a few minutes and then enter dream sleep. Dream sleep is also termed rapid eye movement (REM) sleep, because our eyes move around rapidly while we dream.

The brain and body are quite active while we dream. For instance, heart rate, blood pressure, and breathing rate escalate during dreaming. Our brainwaves also accelerate and blood flow to the brain rises dramatically.

We cannot move when we dream because our large body muscles are paralyzed, apparently so that we can't act out our dreams.

The Purpose of REM Sleep – Mental and Emotional Restoration

The primary functions of dream sleep are to process emotional material and save information in memory, particularly information learned over the latter portion of each day.

REM Brainwaves

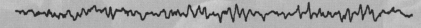

Awake Brainwaves

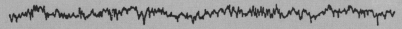

DRUGS AND
HERBS

section 4

DRUGS

As a response to the prevalence of sleep problems in society, drug and herbal sleep remedies have skyrocketed in popularity. The following may help shed light on the most popular aids.

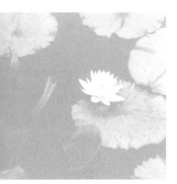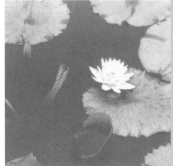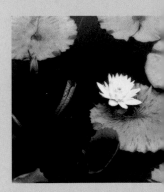

Prescription Sleeping Pills

Sleeping pills fail to treat the causes of insomnia. Because they treat only insomnia's symptoms, any improvement in sleep can only be temporary, thereby perpetuating the cycle of insomnia and sleeping pills.

Like most medicines, sleeping pills can be of short-term value if they are used judiciously. Occasional use of a sleeping pill for a few nights may be appropriate if sleep is temporarily disturbed by jet lag or a stressful event such as the death of a loved one, divorce, or a medical problem. In these circumstances, sleeping pills may help prevent short-term insomnia from evolving into chronic insomnia.

Over-the-Counter Pills

Insomniacs spend more than $100 million annually on over-the-counter sleep aids. A few of the most recognized names include: Sominex, Unisom, Sleep-Eze, Nytol, Tylenol PM, Bufferin Nite-time, Anacin PM, and Excedrin PM.

music instantly

rearranges the

molecular structure

of the body

- carlos santana

Despite all the advertising claims made for these over-the-counter medications, there is virtually no scientific evidence that they are more effective than sugar pills.

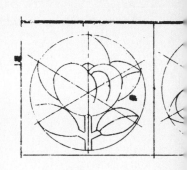

NATURAL AND HERBAL REMEDIES

Although some people find that natural and herbal remedies are effective as a sleep aids, others find that they have little or no effect. Almost no sound scientific research has been done to support these products' claims, and scant information exists concerning their long-term side effects on health.

While there may be benefits associated with certain herbal and natural remedies, they fail to treat the causes of insomnia and reinforce dependency on external agents. If you experiment with herbal remedies, I encourage you to cross-reference several sources that provide information on these substances. Your local health food store and library should have books on natural and herbal sleep remedies.

Please consider the following information regarding melatonin, which has recently become one of the most popular "sleep solution" products.

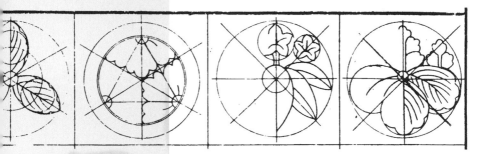

MELATONIN

Sleep experts have concluded that supplemental melatonin has little value in the treatment of insomnia. Scientists also have concerns about melatonin's side effects. It may constrict blood vessels and therefore should not be used by those with heart problems. In high doses, melatonin also inhibits fertility and should not be used by women who are trying to conceive. In fact, melatonin is being tested widely in the Netherlands as a contraceptive. Ironically, sleepiness is not a commonly reported side effect, which casts further doubt on its use as a sleeping pill.

THE ANTI-SLEEP
VIRUS

section 5

Scientists recently have discovered a viral-like sleep killer that can seriously disrupt sleep and also cause or exacerbate many other health problems. This anti-sleep virus compromises the immune system and may even shorten our lifespans.

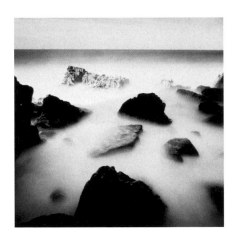

It spreads through the air and is highly contagious. It has been found to infect most of its victims in the workplace, where it seems to spread most effectively.

With documented cases reported in more than 39 countries, this viral-like sleep killer has reached epidemic status.

It is called the Stress Response.

THE STRESS RESPONSE

The Stress Response is a set of involuntary physiological changes that occur in the mind and body whenever we are faced with a 'threatening' situation. It is a survival mechanism that was designed to assist our ancestors in fighting or fleeing acute, well-defined physical threats such as predators. These physical stressors were encountered infrequently, but they were intense and required physical exertion.

TIMES HAVE CHANGED

Since we no longer hunt and gather on a daily basis, we rarely encounter these ancient physical stressors. Instead, our lives today are filled with psychological stressors on our brains that are less intense but more chronic and frequent including: work, traffic, relationships, family and money concerns.

The result is chronic, inappropriate, excessive activation of the Stress Response. For many, the Stress Response occurs so often in daily life that it has become automatic and unconscious.

...by a sleep to

say we end the

heartache and

the thousand

natural shocks

that flesh is

heir to, 'tis a

consummation

devoutly to be

wished...to

sleep...perchance

to dream...

- shakespeare

THE BAD NEWS

Our minds and our bodies treat psychological stress ('mind' stress) and physical stress ('body' stress) very differently.

Although the brain automatically counteracts body stressors by eliciting a relaxation response, the brain does NOT elicit a relaxation response to mind stressors.

For that reason, the repetitive, unending mind stressors that we face each day build and build without a natural counteracting effect to relieve our bodies and our brains.

THE GOOD NEWS

Our brains can be taught to combat mind stress. You can counteract mind stress by consciously eliciting a response that relaxes your brain and body – the Relaxation Response (RR).

The RR is an inborn, quieting response that is elicited by muscular relaxation, mental focusing and breathing techniques.

and the night

shall be filled

with music,

and the cares,

that infest

the day, shall

fold their

tents, like

the arabs, and

as silently

steal away.

- longfellow

The RR is effective in counteracting the Stress Response by relaxing the body and the mind. The relaxing effects of the RR also produce physiological changes that promote sleep, including:

z   *Slower brainwave patterns and mental quieting*

z   *Reductions in heart and breathing rates*

z   *Relaxation of the muscles in the body*

z   *Reduced secretion of stress hormones*

RR AND SLEEP

When you are stressed during the day, your stress hormones are not only elevated during the day; they also are elevated while you sleep.

Dozens of scientific studies have proven that the RR is an effective treatment for insomnia. Daytime practice of the RR improves sleep because it counters daily Stress Responses, and reduces the likelihood that stress hormones will be elevated at night. The RR also improves sleep because it helps turn off negative thoughts – quieting the mind and relaxing the body.

● **Discoveries**

Dr. Herbert Benson was the first to discover the **Relaxation Response** in the 1970's, and his book **"The Relaxation Response"** was on the New York Times Best Seller list with over four million copies sold.

Our recent study at Harvard Medical School suggests that the RR produces a brainwave pattern similar to Stage 1 sleep. Recall that Stage 1 is the transition state between waking and sleeping, characterized by "theta" brainwaves. By practicing the RR at bedtime or after a nighttime awakening, it is easier to enter Stage 1 sleep and ultimately Stage 2, deep sleep, and dream sleep.

LEARNING TO ELICIT THE RR

There are several scientifically proven methods to elicit the Relaxation Response:

z   *Muscular relaxation techniques*

z   *Breathing techniques*

z   *Mental repetition of a word, sound or phrase*

z   *Listening to relaxing music*

While all of these are effective on their own, we have created an exercise that combines all of them together. Details can be found on the following page.

o magic sleep!

o comfortable

bird, that broodiest

o'er the troubled

sea of the mind

till it is hushed

and smooth!

- keats

THE RR EXERCISE

Step 1 - Find a quiet, private place where you can sit or lay down and not be disturbed.

Step 2 - Play Blue Marble's Deep Sleep 101 CD or other relaxing music.

Step 3 - Consciously feel the muscles throughout your body relax. This is accomplished by closing your eyes, then feeling relaxation gradually spread throughout your body. Silently talking yourself through this process usually helps (i.e. "I feel my toes becoming very relaxed/warm/heavy."). Starting with the feet, feeling relaxation spread up to the head seems to work best. Feelings of relaxation may vary from warmth, heaviness, tingling or floating to nothing specific.

Step 4 - Establish a relaxed, deep breathing pattern.

Step 5 - Direct your attention from everyday thoughts by using a mental focusing device that is neutral and repetitive: a word such as one, relax, peace or heavy, or any word you choose. Or, focus on the rise and fall of the abdomen as you breathe. For many, it is helpful to repeat a word silently with each exhalation. In meditation, this is called a "mantra". If your thoughts return to everyday concerns, this is normal, but gently let those thoughts vanish and redirect your focus to your mantra.

It is best to elicit the RR for about 10 to 20 minutes per day. More is fine, and you may find that 30 to 45 minutes provide a very deep state of relaxation and awareness.

DEEP BREATHING 101

When relaxed or sleeping, we breathe with the abdomen, which relaxes the body because carbon dioxide is expelled and oxygen inhaled efficiently. Under stress, we tend to breathe using short and shallow breaths, regular chest breaths, or we hold our breath. We don't inhale oxygen and exhale carbon dioxide effectively, which stresses the body and makes us feel more anxious.

TECHNIQUES THAT PROMOTE
SLEEP

section 6

1. EXERCISE THE BODY

A lack of physical activity can contribute to poor sleep by inhibiting the daily rise and fall of the body-temperature rhythm. In fact, research shows that insomniacs lead more sedentary lives than good sleepers.

When I speak of "exercise", please understand that I do not mean an exhaustive workout in a health club.

> *While big biceps or a flat stomach might be aesthetically appealing, the real purpose of exercise is to produce a physiological state that makes our bodies and our minds feel relaxed and energetic.*

Exercise improves sleep by producing a significant rise in body temperature, followed by a compensatory drop a few hours later.

The drop in body temperature, which persists for two to four hours after exercise, makes it easier to fall asleep and stay asleep.

Exercise also improves sleep because it is a physical stressor to the body. The brain compensates for physical stress by increasing deep sleep.

The beneficial effect of exercise on sleep is greatest when exercise occurs within three to six hours of bedtime. Exercising fewer than three hours before bedtime, however, can make it more difficult to fall asleep, because the body's temperature may be too elevated at bedtime.

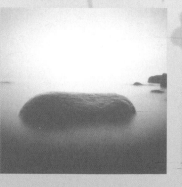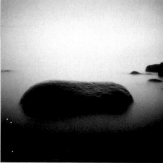

Walking — The Best Exercise Recommendation

I recommend that my patients walk 30 minutes at a brisk pace in bright sunlight each morning or evening. This is a powerful recommendation for improved sleep. Aside from the many other benefits of exercise, a daily brisk walk creates a rise and fall of body temperature that is essential for good sleep. If you are able to walk in bright sunlight, it also provides exposure to bright daylight, which is an essential timing mechanism for sleep.

Yoga — The Other Best Exercise Recommendation

Yoga is effective at both exercising the body and quieting the mind. Once you get beyond the funny name, yoga is simply an age-old technique of stretching, strengthening and relaxing the mind and body.

There are many types of yoga workouts. Depending on the type of yoga session, it can be used as exercise or a relaxation technique.

...keep a bower

quiet for us,

and a sleep

full of sweet

dreams, and

health, and

quiet breathing.

— keats

2. EXPOSE YOURSELF TO SUNLIGHT

The advent of modern technology has significantly altered our exposure to light and darkness. Studies have shown that, no matter where people live, they obtain only one hour of sunlight on average during the day.

The main reason we obtain so little sunlight is that most of us work indoors. A brightly lit room has about 500 luxes of light (a lux is the equivalent of the light from one candle) compared to 10,000 luxes at sunrise and 100,000 at noon on a summer day. To the brain, spending the day indoors is equivalent to spending the day in darkness!

Because sunlight causes body temperature to rise, increasing our exposure to bright natural light and true darkness optimizes our natural melatonin secretion and our body-temperature rhythm to promote effective sleep.

Exposure to sunlight has also been shown to improve mood.

3. WIND DOWN (ONE HOUR BEFORE BEDTIME)

Winding down gradually in the hour before bedtime is helpful in inducing sleep. During this wind-down period, avoid stimulating activities such as telephone calls, arguments or emotional discussions, work-related activities, computers, bill-paying, or unpleasant television programs.

Try any of the following:

Music - As discussed previously, relaxing music is especially effective in quieting the mind and body and it can be combined with another relaxation method. You can use music to enhance any of the following techniques.

Take a Hot Bath - A hot bath causes a rise and fall in body temperature that can make it easier to fall asleep and stay asleep. The bath must be hot and kept hot for about 25 minutes. Also, the bath should be taken about two hours before bedtime to generate the timing for your drop in body temperature.

Yoga as Relaxation - A relaxation-oriented Yoga routine can be tremendously helpful for quieting the mind and body.

4. RELAX AND EXERCISE THE BRAIN

As described in section 5 of this book, psychological stress has become one of the primary causes of poor sleep. At the very least, it is near the top of the list for most individuals experiencing sleep difficulties. Thus, the recommendation to "Create the RR in the Brain" below is one of the most important recommendations in this book.

Create the RR in the brain - See details on pages 20 to 23.

Exercise the brain - Bored people don't sleep very well. Studies have shown that mental and intellectual stimulation during the day increases the pressure for sleep.

...the innocent sleep, sleep that knits up the raveled sleave of care, the death of each day's life, sore labor's bath, balm of hurt minds, great nature's second course, chief nourisher in life's feast. — Shakespeare

5. MAKE YOUR BED AND BEDROOM A CUE FOR SLEEP

Step 1 Use the bedroom for sleep and sexual activity only. Do not use the bedroom to watch television, work, study, or talk on the telephone.

Step 2 Since your goal is to associate the bed with sleep, make sure you feel drowsy when you turn off the lights to go to sleep.

Step 3 If you don't fall asleep within 20 to 30 minutes, or if you awaken during the night and don't fall back to sleep within that time, don't lie in bed tossing and turning. Instead, go to another room or sit up in bed and engage in a quiet, relaxing activity such as reading a book or magazine until you are drowsy, then attempt to go to sleep again. Repeat this process as often as necessary until you fall asleep.

Step 4 Keep your bedroom cool, as a warm room tends to prevent your body temperature from falling (which promotes sleep).

Step 5 Keep your bedroom quiet. All sounds (other than 'white' noise) prevent us from entering deep sleep. Even music played while we sleep tends to prevent us from entering deep sleep.

edgar allen poe said

that sleep is "house

cleaning time...

it's strengthening

things that need

to be strengthened,

weakening things

that no longer

need to be there,

throwing them away."

30

6. SLEEP-SCHEDULING TIPS:

z Get out of bed around the same time every day, including weekends, no matter how little or how poorly you have slept.

z Reduce your time in bed so that it more closely matches the amount of sleep you are getting per night. Reducing time in bed is only temporary until your sleep efficiency improves to 85 percent (you are asleep 85 percent of the time you are in bed).

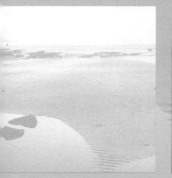
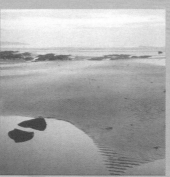
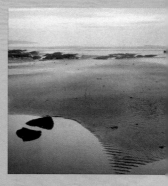

7. LIMIT YOUR INTAKE OF ANTI-SLEEP CHEMICALS

Caffeine

Caffeine is a stimulant that speeds up brainwaves, increases heart rate and blood pressure, promotes alertness and reduces fatigue. These stimulant effects, which work in as little as 15 minutes and can last for six or more hours, can also disturb sleep.

Drinking one or two cups of coffee in the morning is unlikely to affect nighttime sleep. However, coffee should be avoided after lunchtime.

As final words of caution about caffeine: make sure your children don't drink beverages containing caffeine in the afternoon. When a child drinks a can of cola, the caffeine intake is comparable to four cups of coffee for an adult. As a result, your child may not be able to fall asleep at night.

Nicotine

Nicotine also harms sleep. The effects of nicotine are similar to those of caffeine, including faster brainwaves, heart rate and breathing rate, as well as increased amounts of stress hormones.

These stimulant effects, which last for several hours after smoking a cigarette, can make it harder to fall asleep and stay asleep.

Smoking also irritates the upper air passage, which can exacerbate snoring and diminish sleep quality. That's why smokers sleep more poorly than nonsmokers and why insomnia ranks as one of the major health complaints of smokers. In short, smokers cannot expect to sleep well.

Alcohol

As alcohol is metabolized during sleep, it produces mild withdrawal symptoms that cause sleep to become interrupted, shortened, and fragmented. This process suppresses both deep sleep and dream sleep. The body requires about 1.5 hours to metabolize one ounce of alcohol; the mild withdrawal effects last for another two to four hours. This means that a glass of wine with dinner probably will not affect sleep. However, one ounce of alcohol within two hours of bedtime or more than one ounce after dinner probably will cause sleep disruptions.

● Pavlov's Relaxing Ritual. One hour before bedtime, fix a cup of Chamomile tea as you listen to 'Having a Good Time' (the first song on Deep Sleep 101'). Pretty soon, just fixing a cup of tea will begin to relax you (even at work).

APPENDIX

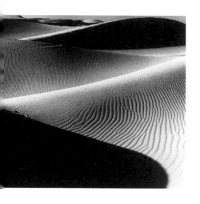

SLEEP DISORDER CENTERS

Sleep disorder centers can fully analyze the many components of breathing, brain activity, muscle movement and even oxygen levels in the body during sleep. If you think you may have a sleep disorder that cannot be cured with the steps recommended in this book, I suggest that you see your physician about an assessment at a sleep disorder clinic.

WHERE TO GO

The American Sleep Disorders Association (ASDA) is the sleep industry's trade group and certification authority. ASDA's website lists the contact information for all accredited sleep disorder clinics in the United States at www.asda.org.

In addition, we have found www.sleepquest.com to be an excellent source for information on sleep and sleep disorders.

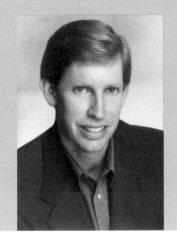

Gregg D. Jacobs, Ph.D., is an Assistant Professor of Psychiatry at Harvard Medical School and a Senior Research Scientist with the Mind/Body Medical Institute of Harvard Medical School. He is credited with developing the world's first drug-free program scientifically proven to conquer insomnia.

GREGG D. JACOBS, PH.D.

PHOTOGRAPHY CREDITS

MUSIC SELECTION: DENNIS CONSTANTINE AND JODY DENBERG

EDITORS: JANE TANNER, KAROL STONE, JENNIFER ABBOTT,
JOY PIERSON AND SUSAN PRIDDY

MUSIC LICENSING AND MANUFACTURING: UNIVERSAL MUSIC GROUP

While pensive poets painful vigils keep, Sleepless themselves to give their readers sleep.

- Alexander Pope

PRODUCED BY: STEVE STONE   DESIGN: GILES DESIGN INC.

MUSIC CREDITS

1. SAMITE
Having A Good Time - 6:05
Written by Samite.
℗ 1999 Windham Hill Records a unit of Windham Hill Music.
Under License from BMG Special Products

2. WIND MACHINE
A Distant Star - 3:07
Written by Steve Mesple.
℗ 1997 Moulin D'Or Recordings.
Courtesy of Moulin D'Or Recordings

3. CHRIS BOTTI
The Steps of Positano - 3:40
Written by Chris Botti.
℗ 1997 The Verve Music Group,
a Division of UMG Recordings, Inc.

4. ROBBIE ROBERTSON & THE RED ROAD ENSEMBLE
The Vanishing Breed - 4:39
Written by Spotted Eagle/Robertson.
℗ 1994 Capitol Records, Inc.
Courtesy Capitol Records,
Under License from EMI-Capitol Music Special Markets

5. BILL FRISELL
Godson Song - 4:38
Written by Bill Frisell.
℗ 1998 Nonesuch Records.
Produced Under License From Atlantic Recording Corp.

6. BOBBY McFERRIN
Common Threads - 4:18
Written by Bobby McFerrin.
℗ 1990 EMI Records. Courtesy EMI Records,
Under License from EMI-Capitol Music Special Markets

7. ULF WAKENIUS/LARS DANIELSSON
Hymn - 4:07
Written by Lars Danielsson.
℗ 1995 Dragon. Courtesy of Dragon

8. PINK MARTINI
Lullaby - 2:12
Written by China Forbes/Thomas M. Lauderdale.
℗ 1997 Heinz Records.
Courtesy of Heinz Records.

9. BUDAPEST STRINGS
Kinderszenen (Scenes from Childhood), Op. 15 – Träumerei – 3:03
Written by Robert Schumann.
℗ 1990 Delta Entertainment Corporation.
Courtesy of Delta Entertainment Corporation,
Los Angeles, California 90025

10. THE CHOIR OF KING'S COLLEGE, CAMBRIDGE -
Ave verum corpus, K.618 - 3:34
Written by Wolfgang Amadeus Mozart.
℗ 1998 Decca Music Group Limited.

11. THE ACADEMY OF ANCIENT MUSIC /WINCHESTER
"Laudate Dominum" from Vesperae Solennes de Confessore - 4:26
Written by Wolfgang Amadeus Mozart.
℗ 1993 Decca Music Group Limited.

12. CLAUDIO ARRAU, piano
Kinderszenen, Op. 15 "Träumerei" - 3:02
Written by Robert Schumann.
℗ 1977 Philips Classics Productions.

13. JULIAN LLOYD WEBBER, cello/JOHN LENEHAN, piano
Wiegenlied, "Cradle Song", Op. 49 No. 4 – 2:32
Written by: Johannes Brahms, arranged by Julian Lloyd Webber.
℗ 1995 Philips Classics Productions.

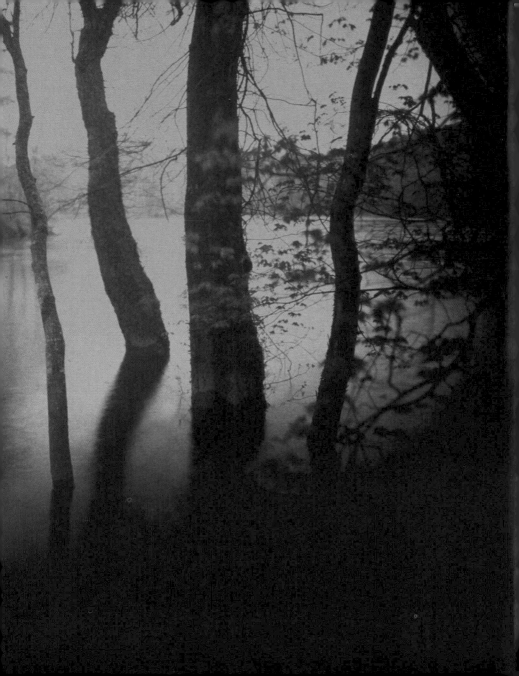